His Majesty's Service

Special Edition

The Caregiver's Daily Journal & Planner

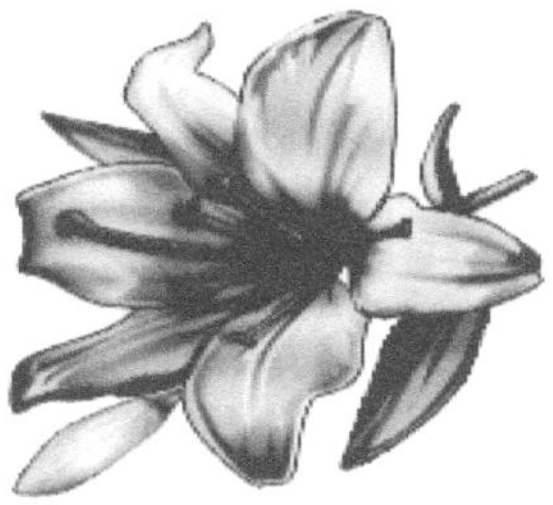

With

Dr. G Landry

His Majesty's Service - Special Edition
The Caregiver's Daily Journal & Planner

ISBN-13: 978-0615685410
ISBN-10: 0615685412

Vienna Schilling Books
Fair Oaks, California
www.viennaschilling.us

Printed in the United States of America

Inside this Special Edition

You'll find ...

A Daily Journal & Planner

A place to list your favorite birthdays and anniversaries

Important Telephone Numbers

Biblical Help Wherever You Are

And the 1-Year Bible Reading Schedule

Use this Daily Journal & Planner alongside

Dr. Landry's charming new book ...

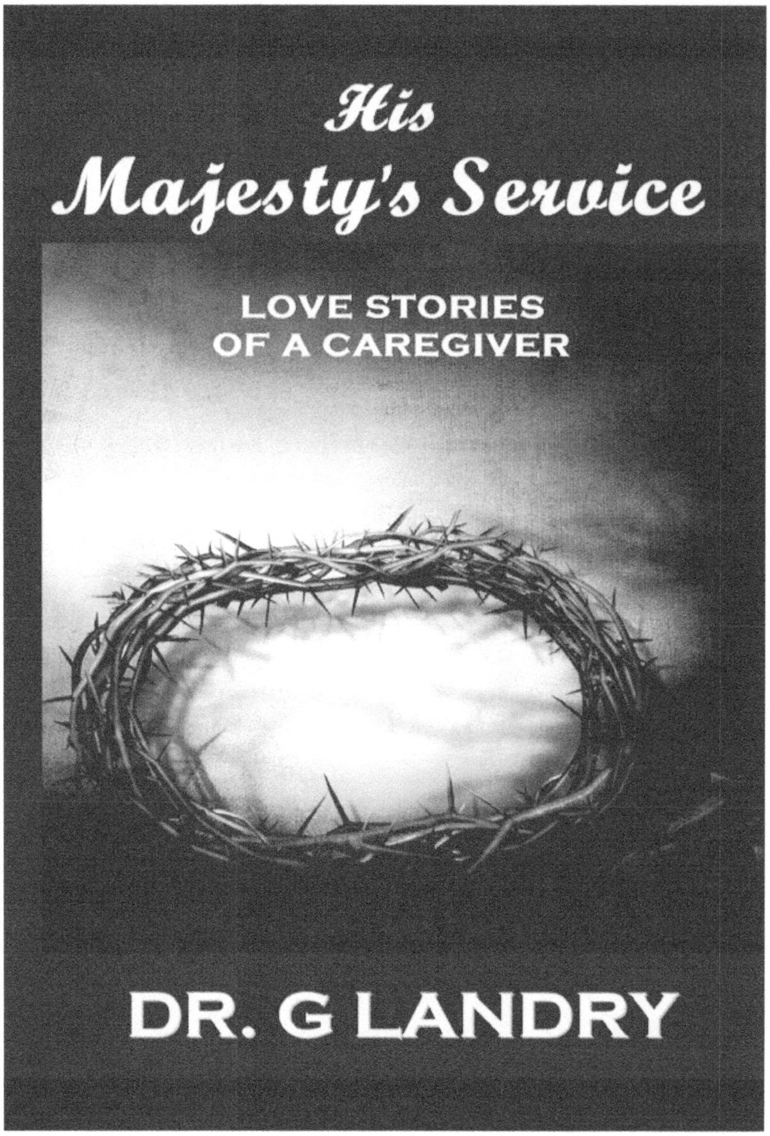

If you haven't already done so, pick up a copy today!

Go to: www.caregiversspeaks.org

Table of Contents

Introduction

When God first called me to be a caregiver many decades ago, I had no idea there even was such a thing. Back in the day, we just did what we had to do to assist our loved ones and neighbors, but times have progressed. Someone came up with another name for 'love' and now it's called 'care-giving.'

Care-giving is defined as: *a family member or paid helper who regularly takes care of a child, sick person, the elderly, or disabled.* Personally, I believe it's the love you share with another.

Recent facts show that 61% of caregivers are women and most are middle-aged. The stress that caregivers carry can be very emotional and many times becomes a tangible, physical strain. Hence, they need ways to unload, even if it's just for an hour a day. Hence, I developed this caregivers' journal for the express purpose of taking us to that place of refreshment.

I found over the years that it helps *immensely* when caregivers come together and *just talk!* Talking about it relieves all kinds of stress we carry from day to day. One way to 'talk about it' is to keep a journal; one that keeps us in touch with priorities, gets us organized, refreshed and ready for each day.

That's why I invite you to join me inside this 4-year journal as we take on the professional art of care-giving, and make a difference in the lives we care for.

I would also like to invite you to become a valued member of our caregivers' group, ***Caregivers Speak***. We meet every week and it's free to join. For times and locations, write us at:

glandrybook@gmail.com

As the founder of ***Caregivers Speak,*** I started the group to provide us with a place where we can come and talk, laugh, fellowship and cry if we like! ***Caregivers Speak*** is a place where no one ever holds anything against us; a place where we can be pampered, recognized and loved. ***Caregivers Speak*** is a place where you can recharge your battery and start fresh! We promise you a wonderful time and you'll look forward to each and every meeting.

In the meantime, we've got this wonderful journal. Know that each day as you interact inside these pages, hundreds of other caregivers across the country are doing the same. If ever there was a fellow-ship 'in the spirit' – this is it; and it's all ours!

I invite you to come and join us at a ***Caregivers Speak*** meeting very soon! Seating is limited, so please send us an email to reserve your seat. For additional copies of this journal and my book entitled 'His Majesty's Service' visit our website at:

www.caregiversspeaks.org

Be blessed & stay strong!
Dr. G Landry

The Caregiver's Daily Journal & Planner

January 1 **Deuteronomy 11:1**

Deuteronomy 10:19 **January 2**

January 3 **Matthew 5:44**

Matthew 22:37-39 **January 4**

January 5 **John 13:34**

John 15:12-13 **January 6**

January 7 **John 13:1**

John 14:21 **January 8**

January 9 **Psalm 5:11**

Psalm 97:10 **January 10**

January 11 **Psalm 17:6**

Isaiah 54:8 **January 12**

January 13 **Nehemiah 9:16-17**

Psalm 36:10 **January 14**

January 15 **Isaiah 54:10**

Psalm 36:7 **January 16**

January 17 **Isaiah 63:7**

Acts 16:31 **January 18**

January 19 **Ephesians 2:7-8**

2nd Samuel 2:6 **January 20**

January 21 **Luke 11:35**

Matthew 5:3 **January 22**

January 23 **Matthew 5:4**

Matthew 5:5 **January 24**

January 25 **Matthew 5:6**

Matthew 5:7 **January 26**

January 27 **Matthew 5:8**

Matthew 5:9 **January 28**

January 29 **Matthew 5:10**

Matthew 5:11 **January 30**

January 31 **Matthew 5:12**

PERSONAL MONTHLY REFLECTIONS

February 1 **Proverbs 15:16**

John 13:34 **February 2**

February 3 **Psalm 51:1**

Psalm 51:2 **February 4**

February 5 **Psalm 51:3**

Psalm 51:4 **February 6**

February 7 **Psalm 51:5**

Psalm 51:6 **February 8**

February 9 **Psalm 51:7**

Psalm 51:8 **February 10**

February 11 **Psalm 51:9**

Psalm 51:10 **February 12**

February 13 **Psalm 51:11**

Psalm 51:12 **February 14**

February 15 **Psalm 55:1**

Psalm 55:2 **February 16**

February 17 **Psalm 55:16-17**

Psalm 92:1 **February 18**

February 19 **Psalm 92:2**

Psalm 143:6 **February 20**

February 21 **Psalm 143:7**

Psalm 143:8 **February 22**

February 23 **Psalm 143:9**

Psalm 143:9 **February 24**

February 25 **Psalm 143:10**

Psalm 143:11 **February 26**

February 27 **Psalm 143:12**

Psalm 145:1 **February 28**

PERSONAL MONTHLY REFLECTIONS:

March 1

Ephesians 6:5

Romans 13:8

March 2

March 3

Romans 14:13

1st Corinthians 13:1

March 4

March 5

1st Corinthians 13:2

1st Corinthians 13:3

March 6

March 7

1st Corinthians 13:4

Psalm 105:14

March 8

March 9 **Psalm 105:15**

Jeremiah 30:17 **March 10**

March 11

Matthew 7:1

Matthew 7:2

March 12

March 13

Matthew 7:3

Matthew 7:4

March 14

March 15

James 5:14

March 16

James 5:15

March 17

James 5:16

2nd Kings 20:4-5

March 18

March 19

Psalm 103:1

Psalm 103:2

March 20

March 21

Psalm 103:3

Psalm 103:4

March 22

March 23

Psalm 103:5

Psalm 103:6

March 24

March 25

Jude 21

Revelation 2:11

March 26

March 27

2nd Chronicles 20:17

Isaiah 54:17

March 28

March 29

John 9:11

1st Timothy 6:17

March 30

March 31

Psalm 119:149

PERSONAL MONTHLY REFLECTIONS:

April 1

Proverbs 19:17

Jeremiah 17:14

April 2

April 3

Matthew 6:1

Matthew 6:4

April 4

April 5

2nd Corinthians 9:6

1st Peter 5:7

April 6

April 7

Isaiah 43:19

Nehemiah 8:10

April 8

April 9

Luke 6:38

Isaiah 40:31

April 10

April 11

Proverbs 16:3

1st Corinithians 15:57

April 12

April 13

Psalm 59:1-2

Psalm 84:11

April 14

April 15

Psalm 44:3

Ephesians 2:7

April 16

April 17

Isaiah 62:6-7

Proverbs 31:28

April 18

April 19

Psalm 46:1

Genesis 12:2

April 20

April 21

Psalm 75:10

Psalm 8:5

April 22

April 23

Job 33:26

Ephesian 4:26

April 24

April 25

2nd Timothy 3:16

Habakkuk 3:18

April 26

April 27

Matthew 12:18

Luke 12:32

April 28

April 29

Matthew 6:33

Leviticus 26:9-10

April 30

PERSONAL MONTHLY REFLECTIONS:

May 1

2nd Chronicles 20:17

Psalm 27:1

May 2

May 3

Ecclesiastes 3:1

Isaiah 10:27

May 4

May 5

Isaiah 26:3-4

Jeremiah 42:10

May 6

May 7

Lamentations 3:26

Amos 9:15

May 8

May 9

Joel 2:25-26

Hosea 3:6

May 10

May 11

Daniel 9:18

Ezekiel 3:22

May 12

May 13

Jonah 3:1-2

Lamentations 3:23

May 14

May 15

Micah 4:5

Zephaniah 3:15

May 16

May 17

Haggai 1:5

Zechariah 8:17

May 18

May 19

Matthew 4:4

Lamentations 3:60

May 20

May 21

Malachi 3:10

Zechariah 8:12

May 22

May 23

Lamentations 3:24

Matthew 6:15

May 24

May 25

Lamentations 3:25

Matthew 6:2

May 26

May 27

Lamentations 3:58

Lamentations 3:57

May 28

May 29

Matthew 7:1

Matthew 6:41

May 30

May 31

Mark 9:41

PERSONAL MONTHLY REFLECTIONS:

June 1

Mark 11:25

John 8:36

June 2

June 3

Acts 13:47

Romans 6:23

June 4

June 5

Romans 6:12

Romans 8:39

June 6

June 7

Romans 13:8

2nd Corinthians 9:7

June 8

June 9

2nd Thessalonians 3:3

1st Timothy 5:1-2

June 10

June 11

2nd Timothy 1:7

Revelation 1:18

June 12

June 13

Proverbs 4:23

Psalm 22:10

June 14

June 15

Psalm 5:12

Nehemiah 1:9

June 16

June 17

James 5:16

Titus 3:5

June 18

June 19

1st Corinthians 13:4

Psalm 140:1

June 20

June 21

Psalm 119:169

Psalm 37: 3

June 22

June 23

Psalm 23:1

Proverbs 3:5

June 24

June 25

Isaiah 1:19

Genesis 39:21

June 26

June 27

Deuteronomy 28:7

Joshua 1:6

June 28

June 29

Joshua 1:8

June 30

Ruth 1:16

PERSONAL MONTHLY REFLECTIONS:

July 1

2nd Kings 20:5

1st Peter 2:2

July 2

July 3

2nd Corinthians 12:10

Isaiah 26:3

July 4

July 5

1st Thessaians 3:8

Matthew 7:24

July 6

July 7

Joshua 24:15

Job 42:1-2

July 8

July 9

Psalm 18:29-30

James 1:2

July 10

July 11

Proverbs 16:17-18

1st Peter 2:11

July 12

July 15

2nd Corinthians 5:20

Proverbs 18:21

July 16

July 17

Proverbs 16:19

Ephesians 5:2

July 18

July 19

2nd Corinthians 12:10

Hebrews 12:1-2

July 20

July 21

Mark 13:13

July 22

Ecclesiastes 9:7

July 23

Genesis 39:21

Esther 2:17

July 24

July 25

Deuteronomy 11:28

1st Peter 5:6

July 26

July 27

Palms 34:1

Genesis 50:20

July 28

July 29

Hebrews 12:3

Psalms 34:18

July 30

July 31

Matthew 10:10

PERSONAL MONTHLY REFLECTIONS:

August 1

2nd Corinthians 3:2

Ephesians 1:6

August 2

August 3

Hebrews 11:1

Galatians 3:14

August 4

August 5

Luke 16;12

Matthew 6:20

August 6

August 7

Proverbs 27:20

Philippians 4:11-12

August 8

August 9

Philippians 3:13

Philippians 3:14

August 10

August 11

Matthew 5:1

2nd Kings 4:26

August 12

August 13

Romans 16:17

1st Corinthians 5:11

August 14

August 15

1st Corinthians 15:33

Amos 3:3

August 16

August 17

Matthew 5:19

Ecclesiastes 1:8

August 18

August 19

Ecclesiastes 1:9

Ecclesiastes 1:10

August 20

August 21

Isaiah 62:6

Isaiah 62:7

August 22

August 23

Jeremiah 4:2

Daniel 2:23

August 24

August 25

Amos 7:15

Zephaniah 3:12

August 26

August 27

Zephaniah 3:20

Haggai 1:5

August 28

August 29

Matthew 13:23

John 3:11

August 30

August 31

John 3:16

PERSONAL MONTHLY REFLECTIONS:

September 1

Colossians 1:3

Philemon 4

September 2

September 3

Hebrews 10:9

Revelation 2:11

September 4

September 5

James 5:7

1st Peter 1:3

September 6

September 7

James 1:3

September 8

James 4:10

September 9

2nd Corinthians 4:18

September 10

Luke 11:35

September 11

Ezekiel 28:20-21

Psalm 91:1

September 12

September 13

Psalm 40:1

Psalm 39:1

September 14

September 15

Psalm 37:3

Psalm 37:34

September 16

September 17

Psalm 26:1-3

Psalm 23:4

September 18

September 19

Matthew 6:33

Nehemiah 1:9

September 20

September 21

1st Samuel 30:8

Exodus 14:14

September 22

September 23

John 10:13

Psalm 104:1

September 24

September 25

John 6:27

Luke 12:22

September 26

September 27

September 28

September 29

Matthew 6:25

Luke 12:7

September 30

PERSONAL MONTHLY REFLECTIONS:

October 1

Proverb 16:3

Deuteronomy 7:9

October 2

October 3

Deuteronomy 10:18

Jeremiah 31:3

October 4

October 5

John 3:16

2nd Corinthians 9:7

October 6

October 7

Ephesians 2:4

1st John 3:2

October 8

October 9

1st John 4:1

Song of Solomon 1:4

October 10

October 11

Matthew 17:7

1st Timothy 2:2-3

October 12

October 13

Psalm 107:43

John 11:5

October 14

October 15

John 14:31

October 16

John 15:12

October 17

Deuteronomy 30:20

Matthew 4:4

October 18

October 19

Luke 2:23

Lamentations 3:23

October 20

October 21

Lamentations 3:24

Lamentations 3:25

October 22

October 23

Lamentations 3:26

Lamentations 3:57

October 24

October 25

Isaiah 55:11

Psalm 149:4

October 26

October 27

Psalm 148:5

Psalm 1:1

October 28

October 29

Job 36:11

October 30

Job 36:12

October 31

Psalm 103:1

PERSONAL MONTHLY REFLECTIONS:

November 1

Psalm 103:2

Psalm 103:3

November 2

November 3

Psalm 101:2

Psalm 102:1

November 4

November 5

Psalm 24:7

Psalm 146:2

November 6

November 7

Psalm 107:43

Genesis 26:3

November 8

November 9

Genesis 26:24

1st Corinthians 3:5

November 10

November 11

Nehemiah 8:10

November 12

Ephesians 6:13

November 13

Isaiah 45:21

Isaiah 43:19

November 14

November 15

Ephesians 4:29

Luke 6:38

November 16

November 17

Psalm 84:11

Ephesians 4:31

November 18

November 19

James 3:16

Isaiah 40:31

November 20

November 21

Leviticus 19:33-34

Jeremiah 6:2

November 22

November 23

Matthew 6:9

Matthew 6:10

November 24

November 25

Matthew 6:11

Matthew 6:12

November 26

November 27

Matthew 6:13

Matthew 6:14

November 28

November 29

Matthew 6:15

Matthew 7:15

November 30

PERSONAL MONTHLY REFLECTIONS:

December 1

Titus 3:1

Titus 3:2

December 2

December 3

Titus 3:5

Acts 7:49

December 4

December 5

Acts 7:50

Galatians 2:20

December 6

December 7

Revelation 14:12

1st John 1:9

December 8

December 9

James 4:6

1st Timothy 6:17

December 10

December 11

Romans 3:23

John 1:51

December 12

December 13

Luke 4:8

Mark 1:2

December 14

December 15

Isaiah 53:5

Psalm 120:1

December 16

December 17

Psalm 122:1

Psalm 105:1

December 18

December 19

Psalm 105:2

Psalm 105:3

December 20

December 21

Psalm 105:4

Psalm 105:5

December 22

December 23

Proverbs 23:7

Psalm 51:2

December 24

December 25

Luke 1:30-31

Ephesians 4:26

December 26

December 27

Ephesians 4:29

Ephesians 4:27

December 28

December 29

Ephesians 4:31

Ephesians 4:32

December 30

December 31

2nd Corinthians 13:11-12

PERSONAL MONTHLY REFLECTIONS:

Birthdays

&

Anniversaries

Birthdays & Anniversaries

January

February

March

April

May

June

July

August

September

October

November

December

Important Telephone Numbers

Name:	Number:

Important Telephone Numbers

Name:	Number:

North American Area Codes

CODE	STATE
205	Alabama
251	Alabama
256	Alabama
334	Alabama
938	Alabama
907	Alaska
684	American Samoa
264	Anguilla
268	Antigua & Barbuda
480	Arizona
520	Arizona
602	Arizona
623	Arizona
928	Arizona
479	Arkansas
501	Arkansas
870	Arkansas
242	Bahamas
246	Barbados
441	Bermuda
284	British Virgin Islands
209	California
213	California
310	California
323	California
408	California
415	California
424	California
442	California
510	California
530	California
559	California
562	California
619	California
626	California
650	California
657	California
661	California

CODE	STATE
707	California
714	California
747	California
760	California
805	California
818	California
831	California
858	California
909	California
916	California
925	California
949	California
951	California
345	Cayman Islands
303	Colorado
719	Colorado
720	Colorado
970	Colorado
203	Connecticut
475	Connecticut
860	Connecticut
302	Delaware
767	Dominica
809	Dominican Republic
829	Dominican Republic
849	Dominican Republic
911	Emergency
239	Florida
305	Florida
321	Florida
352	Florida
386	Florida
407	Florida
561	Florida
727	Florida
754	Florida
772	Florida
786	Florida

CODE	STATE
813	Florida
863	Florida
904	Florida
941	Florida
954	Florida
850	Florida
229	Georgia
404	Georgia
470	Georgia
478	Georgia
678	Georgia
706	Georgia
762	Georgia
770	Georgia
912	Georgia
473	Grenada
671	Guam
808	Hawaii
208	Idaho
217	Illinois
224	Illinois
309	Illinois
312	Illinois
331	Illinois
618	Illinois
630	Illinois
708	Illinois
773	Illinois
779	Illinois
815	Illinois
847	Illinois
872	Illinois
260	Indiana
317	Indiana
765	Indiana
219	Indiana
812	Indiana
574	Indiana
319	Iowa
515	Iowa
563	Iowa

CODE	STATE
641	Iowa
712	Iowa
876	Jamaica
316	Kansas
913	Kansas
620	Kansas
785	Kansas
502	Kentucky
859	Kentucky
270	Kentucky
606	Kentucky
225	Louisiana
318	Louisiana
337	Louisiana
504	Louisiana
985	Louisiana
207	Maine
240	Maryland
301	Maryland
410	Maryland
443	Maryland
339	Massachusetts
351	Massachusetts
413	Massachusetts
508	Massachusetts
617	Massachusetts
774	Massachusetts
781	Massachusetts
857	Massachusetts
978	Massachusetts
231	Michigan
248	Michigan
269	Michigan
313	Michigan
517	Michigan
586	Michigan
616	Michigan
734	Michigan
810	Michigan
947	Michigan
989	Michigan
906	Michigan
218	Minnesota
320	Minnesota
507	Minnesota

CODE	STATE
612	Minnesota
651	Minnesota
763	Minnesota
952	Minnesota
228	Mississippi
601	Mississippi
662	Mississippi
769	Mississippi
314	Missouri
417	Missouri
573	Missouri
636	Missouri
660	Missouri
816	Missouri
406	Montana
664	Montserrat
402	Nebraska
531	Nebraska
308	Nebraska
702	Nevada
775	Nevada
603	New Hampshire
201	New Jersey
551	New Jersey
609	New Jersey
732	New Jersey
848	New Jersey
856	New Jersey
862	New Jersey
908	New Jersey
973	New Jersey
505	New Mexico
575	New Mexico
212	New York
315	New York
347	New York
516	New York
518	New York
585	New York
607	New York
631	New York
646	New York
716	New York
718	New York
845	New York

CODE	STATE
914	New York
917	New York
929	New York
252	North Carolina
336	North Carolina
704	North Carolina
828	No. Carolina
910	No. Carolina
919	No. Carolina
980	No. Carolina
701	North Dakota
670	No. Mariana Island
216	Ohio
234	Ohio
330	Ohio
419	Ohio
440	Ohio
513	Ohio
567	Ohio
614	Ohio
740	Ohio
937	Ohio
405	Oklahoma
539	Oklahoma
580	Oklahoma
918	Oklahoma
458	Oregon
541	Oregon
503	Oregon
971	Oregon
215	Pennsylvania
267	Pennsylvania
412	Pennsylvania
484	Pennsylvania
570	Pennsylvania
610	Pennsylvania
717	Pennsylvania
724	Pennsylvania
814	Pennsylvania
878	Pennsylvania
787	Puerto Rico
939	Puerto Rico
401	Rhode Island
803	South Carolina

CODE	STATE
843	South Carolina
864	South Carolina
605	South Dakota
615	Tennessee
731	Tennessee
901	Tennessee
865	Tennessee
931	Tennessee
423	Tennessee
210	Texas
214	Texas
254	Texas
281	Texas
325	Texas
361	Texas
409	Texas
430	Texas
432	Texas
469	Texas
512	Texas
682	Texas
713	Texas
806	Texas
817	Texas
830	Texas
832	Texas
903	Texas
936	Texas
940	Texas
956	Texas
972	Texas
979	Texas
915	Texas
340	US Virgin Islands
385	Utah
435	Utah
801	Utah
802	Vermont
276	Virginia
434	Virginia
540	Virginia
571	Virginia
703	Virginia
757	Virginia

CODE	STATE
804	Virginia
206	Washington
253	Washington
360	Washington
425	Washington
509	Washington
202	Washington D.C.
304	West Virginia
681	West Virginia
262	Wisconsin
414	Wisconsin
534	Wisconsin
608	Wisconsin
715	Wisconsin
920	Wisconsin
307	Wyoming

International Country Codes

NAME OF COUNTRY	CODE
AFGHANISTAN	93
ALBANIA	355
ALGERIA (El Djazaïr)	213
AMERICAN SAMOA	684
ANDORRA	376
ANGOLA	244
ANGUILLA	264
ANTIGUA AND BARBUDA	268
ARGENTINA	54
ARMENIA	7
ARUBA	297
ASCENSION ISLAND	247
AUSTRALIA	61
AUSTRIA	43
AZERBAIJAN	994
BAHAMAS	242
BAHRAIN	973
BANGLADESH	880
BARBADOS	246
BELARUS	375
BELGIUM	32
BELIZE	501
BENIN	229
BERMUDA	441
BHUTAN	975
BOLIVIA	591
BONAIRE, ST. EUSTATIUS, AND SABA	599
BOSNIA AND HERZEGOVINA	387
BOTSWANA	267
BRAZIL	55
BRUNEI DARUSSALAM	673
BULGARIA	359

NAME OF COUNTRY	CODE
BURKINA FASO	226
BURUNDI	257
CAMBODIA	855
CAMEROON	237
CANADA	1
CAPE VERDE	238
CAYMAN ISLANDS	345
CENTRAL AFRICAN REPUBLIC	236
CHAD (Tchad)	235
CHILE	56
CHINA	86
COLOMBIA	57
COMOROS	269
CONGO, REPUBLIC OF	242-243
COOK ISLANDS	682
COSTA RICA	506
CÔTE D'IVOIRE (Ivory Coast)	225
CROATIA (Hrvatska)	385
CUBA	53
CURAÃ‡AO	599
CYPRUS	357
CZECH REPUBLIC	420
DENMARK	45
DJIBOUTI	253
DOMINICA	767
DOMINICAN REPUBLIC	809
ECUADOR	593
EGYPT	20
EL SALVADOR	503
EQUATORIAL GUINEA	240
ERITREA	291
ESTONIA	372

NAME OF COUNTRY	CODE
ETHIOPIA	251
FAEROE ISLANDS	298
FALKLAND ISLANDS	500
FIJI	679
FINLAND	358
FRANCE	33
FRENCH GUIANA	594
FRENCH POLYNESIA	689
GABON	241
GAMBIA, THE	220
GERMANY (Deutschland)	49
GHANA	233
GIBRALTAR	350
GREAT BRITAIN - U.K..	44
GREECE	30
GREENLAND	299
GRENADA	473
GUADELOUPE	590
GUAM	671
GUATEMALA	502
GUINEA	224
GUINEA-BISSAU	245
GUYANA	592
HAITI	509
HONDURAS	504
HONG KONG (Special Administrative Region of China)	852
HUNGARY	36
ICELAND	354
INDIA	91
INDONESIA	62
IRAN (Islamic Republic of Iran)	98
IRAQ	964
IRELAND	353

NAME OF COUNRY	CODE
ISRAEL	972
ITALY	39
JAMAICA	876
JAPAN	81
JORDAN (Hashemite Kingdom of Jordan)	962
KAZAKHSTAN	7
KENYA	254
KIRIBATI	686
KOREA (Democratic Peoples Republic of [North] Korea)	850
KOREA (Republic of [South] Korea)	82
KUWAIT	965
KYRGYZSTAN	996
LAO PEOPLE'S DEMOCRATIC REPUBLIC	856
LATVIA	371
LEBANON	961
LESOTHO	266
LIBERIA	231
LIBYA (Libyan Arab Jamahirya)	218
LIECHTENSTEIN	423
LITHUANIA	370
LUXEMBOURG	352
MACAO (Special Administrative Region of China)	853
MACEDONIA (Former Yugoslav Republic of Macedonia)	389
MADAGASCAR	261
MALAWI	265
MALAYSIA	60
MALDIVES	960
MALI	223
MALTA	356
MARSHALL ISLANDS	692

NAME OF COUNTRY	CODE
MARTINIQUE	596
MAURITANIA	222
MAURITIUS	230
MAYOTTE	269
MEXICO	52
MICRONESIA (Federated States of Micronesia)	691
MOLDOVA	373
MONACO	377
MONGOLIA	976
MONTENEGRO	382
MONTSERRAT	664
MOROCCO	212
MOZAMBIQUE (Moçam-bique)	258
MYANMAR (formerly Burma)	95
Name of Country	Code
Name of Country	Code
Name of Country	Code
Name of Country	Code
NAMIBIA	264
NAURU	674
NEPAL	977
NETHERLANDS	31
NETHERLANDS ANTILLES (obsolete)	599
NEW CALEDONIA	687
NEW ZEALAND	64
NICARAGUA	505
NIGER	227
NIGERIA	234
NIUE	683
NORTHERN MARIANA ISLANDS	670
NORWAY	47
OMAN	968

NAME OF COUNTRY	CODE
PAKISTAN	92
PALAU	680
PALESTINIAN TERRITORIES	970
PANAMA	507
PAPUA NEW GUINEA	675
PARAGUAY	595
PERU	51
PHILIPPINES	63
POLAND	48
PORTUGAL	351
PUERTO RICO	1
QATAR	974
RÉUNION	262
ROMANIA	40
RUSSIAN FEDERATION	7
RWANDA	250
SAINT HELENA	290
SAINT KITTS AND NEVIS	869
SAINT LUCIA	758
SAINT PIERRE AND MIQUELON	508
SAINT VINCENT AND THE GRENADINES	784
SAMOA (formerly Western Samoa)	685
SAN MARINO (Republic of)	378
SAO TOME AND PRINCIPE	239
SAUDI ARABIA (Kingdom of Saudi Arabia)	966
SENEGAL	221
SERBIA (Republic of Serbia)	381
SEYCHELLES	248
SIERRA LEONE	232
SINGAPORE	65
SINT MAARTEN	599
SLOVAKIA (Slovak Repub-lic)	421

NAME OF COUNTRY	CODE
SLOVENIA	386
SOLOMON ISLANDS	677
SOMALIA	252
SOUTH AFRICA (Zuid Afrika)	27
SPAIN (España)	34
SRI LANKA (formerly Ceylon)	94
SUDAN	249
SURINAME	597
SWAZILAND	268
SWEDEN	46
SWITZERLAND	41
SYRIAN ARAB REPUBLIC	963
TAIWAN ("Chinese Taipei" for IOC)	886
TAJIKISTAN	992
TANZANIA	255
THAILAND	66
TIMOR-LESTE (formerly East Timor)	670
TOGO	228
TOKELAU	690
TONGA	676
TRINIDAD AND TOBAGO	868

NAME OF COUNTRY	CODE
TUNISIA	216
TURKEY	90
TURKMENISTAN	993
TURKS AND CAICOS ISLANDS	649
TUVALU	688
UGANDA	256
UKRAINE	380
UNITED ARAB EMIRATES	971
UNITED KINGDOM	44
UNITED STATES	1
URUGUAY	598
UZBEKISTAN	998
VANUATU	678
VATICAN CITY (Holy See)	379
VENEZUELA	58
VIET NAM	84
VIRGIN ISLANDS, BRITISH	284
VIRGIN ISLANDS, U.S.	340
WALLIS AND FUTUNA	681
YEMEN (Yemen Arab Republic)	967
ZAMBIA (formerly Northern Rhodesia)	260
ZIMBABWE	263

Personal

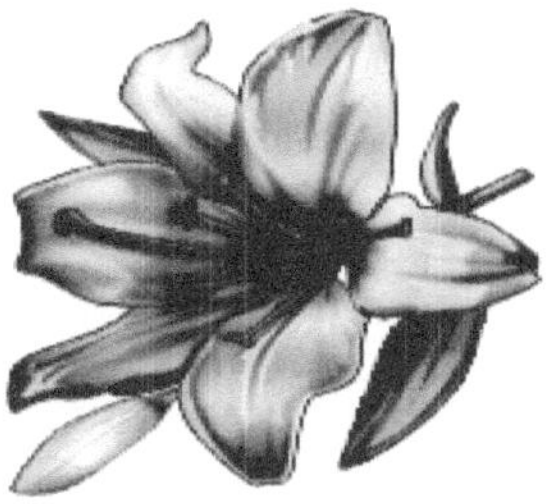

Reflections ...

Personal Reflections

Humane Biblical Laws

Duties Toward Persons

Humane Biblical Laws

Widows and orphans	Exodus 22:22-23
Neighbors	Leviticus 19:13
The poor	Leviticus 19:9-10
Strangers	Leviticus 19:33-34
Needy and helpless	Leviticus 19:14
Servants	Deuteronomy 24:14-15

Duties of the Servant

The definition of a 'servant' is as follows:

Works for a master ... a helper ... slave ... an assistant ... waits on others ... prepares and offers food ... provides guests with comforts, such as food, drink and shelter ... one who hears the call of duty to another ...

Scripture References Defining the Servant

Genesis 24:4-5

Genesis 26

Exodus 14:26-31

Deuteronomy 10:12

2 Samuel 22:44

1 Chronicles 28:9

Proverbs 19:17

Isaiah 41:8-10

Biblical Help Wherever You Are ...

Treatment of Others...	Ephesians 4:32
When Things Look Blue.......................................	Isaiah 40
If You Are Facing A Crisis....................................	Psalm 46
When You Are Discouraged................................	Psalm 23
To Live Successfully With Your Fellow Man....	Romans 12
If You Are Sick and In Pain..................................	Psalm 91
When You Leave Home for Labor or Travel.....	Psalm 121
	Matthew 11:28-30
When You Are Weary..	Romans 8:31-39
If You Have Experienced Severe Loss...............	Romans 8
When You Have Been Placed In A Position of Great Responsibility..	Joshua 1
A Prayer For Forgiveness....................................	Psalm 51
Hope In Time Of Trouble....................................	Psalm 42
For Inward Peace...	John 14

2012 – 2015

Calendar & Notes

2012

January

Su	Mo	Tu	We	Th	Fr	Sa
1	2	3	4	5	6	7
8	9	10	11	12	13	14
15	16	17	18	19	20	21
22	23	24	25	26	27	28
29	30	31				

February

Su	Mo	Tu	We	Th	Fr	Sa
			1	2	3	4
5	6	7	8	9	10	11
12	13	14	15	16	17	18
19	20	21	22	23	24	25
26	27	28	29			

March

Su	Mo	Tu	We	Th	Fr	Sa
				1	2	3
4	5	6	7	8	9	10
11	12	13	14	15	16	17
18	19	20	21	22	23	24
25	26	27	28	29	30	31

April

Su	Mo	Tu	We	Th	Fr	Sa
1	2	3	4	5	6	7
8	9	10	11	12	13	14
15	16	17	18	19	20	21
22	23	24	25	26	27	28
29	30					

May

Su	Mo	Tu	We	Th	Fr	Sa
		1	2	3	4	5
6	7	8	9	10	11	12
13	14	15	16	17	18	19
20	21	22	23	24	25	26
27	28	29	30	31		

June

Su	Mo	Tu	We	Th	Fr	Sa
					1	2
3	4	5	6	7	8	9
10	11	12	13	14	15	16
17	18	19	20	21	22	23
24	25	26	27	28	29	30

July

Su	Mo	Tu	We	Th	Fr	Sa
1	2	3	4	5	6	7
8	9	10	11	12	13	14
15	16	17	18	19	20	21
22	23	24	25	26	27	28
29	30	31				

August

Su	Mo	Tu	We	Th	Fr	Sa
			1	2	3	4
5	6	7	8	9	10	11
12	13	14	15	16	17	18
19	20	21	22	23	24	25
26	27	28	29	30	31	

September

Su	Mo	Tu	We	Th	Fr	Sa
						1
2	3	4	5	6	7	8
9	10	11	12	13	14	15
16	17	18	19	20	21	22
23	24	25	26	27	28	29
30						

October

Su	Mo	Tu	We	Th	Fr	Sa
	1	2	3	4	5	6
7	8	9	10	11	12	13
14	15	16	17	18	19	20
21	22	23	24	25	26	27
28	29	30	31			

November

Su	Mo	Tu	We	Th	Fr	Sa
				1	2	3
4	5	6	7	8	9	10
11	12	13	14	15	16	17
18	19	20	21	22	23	24
25	26	27	28	29	30	

December

Su	Mo	Tu	We	Th	Fr	Sa
						1
2	3	4	5	6	7	8
9	10	11	12	13	14	15
16	17	18	19	20	21	22
23	24	25	26	27	28	29
30	31					

January

February

March

April

May

June

July

August

September

October

November

December

2013

January

Su	Mo	Tu	We	Th	Fr	Sa
		1	2	3	4	5
6	7	8	9	10	11	12
13	14	15	16	17	18	19
20	21	22	23	24	25	26
27	28	29	30	31		

February

Su	Mo	Tu	We	Th	Fr	Sa
					1	2
3	4	5	6	7	8	9
10	11	12	13	14	15	16
17	18	19	20	21	22	23
24	25	26	27	28		

March

Su	Mo	Tu	We	Th	Fr	Sa
					1	2
3	4	5	6	7	8	9
10	11	12	13	14	15	16
17	18	19	20	21	22	23
24	25	26	27	28	29	30
31						

April

Su	Mo	Tu	We	Th	Fr	Sa
	1	2	3	4	5	6
7	8	9	10	11	12	13
14	15	16	17	18	19	20
21	22	23	24	25	26	27
28	29	30				

May

Su	Mo	Tu	We	Th	Fr	Sa
			1	2	3	4
5	6	7	8	9	10	11
12	13	14	15	16	17	18
19	20	21	22	23	24	25
26	27	28	29	30	31	

June

Su	Mo	Tu	We	Th	Fr	Sa
						1
2	3	4	5	6	7	8
9	10	11	12	13	14	15
16	17	18	19	20	21	22
23	24	25	26	27	28	29
30						

July

Su	Mo	Tu	We	Th	Fr	Sa
	1	2	3	4	5	6
7	8	9	10	11	12	13
14	15	16	17	18	19	20
21	22	23	24	25	26	27
28	29	30	31			

August

Su	Mo	Tu	We	Th	Fr	Sa
				1	2	3
4	5	6	7	8	9	10
11	12	13	14	15	16	17
18	19	20	21	22	23	24
25	26	27	28	29	30	31

September

Su	Mo	Tu	We	Th	Fr	Sa
1	2	3	4	5	6	7
8	9	10	11	12	13	14
15	16	17	18	19	20	21
22	23	24	25	26	27	28
29	30					

October

Su	Mo	Tu	We	Th	Fr	Sa
		1	2	3	4	5
6	7	8	9	10	11	12
13	14	15	16	17	18	19
20	21	22	23	24	25	26
27	28	29	30	31		

November

Su	Mo	Tu	We	Th	Fr	Sa
					1	2
3	4	5	6	7	8	9
10	11	12	13	14	15	16
17	18	19	20	21	22	23
24	25	26	27	28	29	30

December

Su	Mo	Tu	We	Th	Fr	Sa
1	2	3	4	5	6	7
8	9	10	11	12	13	14
15	16	17	18	19	20	21
22	23	24	25	26	27	28
29	30	31				

January

February

March

April

May

June

July

August

September

October

November

December

2014

January

Su	Mo	Tu	We	Th	Fr	Sa
			1	2	3	4
5	6	7	8	9	10	11
12	13	14	15	16	17	18
19	20	21	22	23	24	25
26	27	28	29	30	31	

February

Su	Mo	Tu	We	Th	Fr	Sa
						1
2	3	4	5	6	7	8
9	10	11	12	13	14	15
16	17	18	19	20	21	22
23	24	25	26	27	28	

March

Su	Mo	Tu	We	Th	Fr	Sa
						1
2	3	4	5	6	7	8
9	10	11	12	13	14	15
16	17	18	19	20	21	22
23	24	25	26	27	28	29
30	31					

April

Su	Mo	Tu	We	Th	Fr	Sa
		1	2	3	4	5
6	7	8	9	10	11	12
13	14	15	16	17	18	19
20	21	22	23	24	25	26
27	28	29	30			

May

Su	Mo	Tu	We	Th	Fr	Sa
				1	2	3
4	5	6	7	8	9	10
11	12	13	14	15	16	17
18	19	20	21	22	23	24
25	26	27	28	29	30	31

June

Su	Mo	Tu	We	Th	Fr	Sa
1	2	3	4	5	6	7
8	9	10	11	12	13	14
15	16	17	18	19	20	21
22	23	24	25	26	27	28
29	30					

July

Su	Mo	Tu	We	Th	Fr	Sa
		1	2	3	4	5
6	7	8	9	10	11	12
13	14	15	16	17	18	19
20	21	22	23	24	25	26
27	28	29	30	31		

August

Su	Mo	Tu	We	Th	Fr	Sa
					1	2
3	4	5	6	7	8	9
10	11	12	13	14	15	16
17	18	19	20	21	22	23
24	25	26	27	28	29	30
31						

September

Su	Mo	Tu	We	Th	Fr	Sa
	1	2	3	4	5	6
7	8	9	10	11	12	13
14	15	16	17	18	19	20
21	22	23	24	25	26	27
28	29	30				

October

Su	Mo	Tu	We	Th	Fr	Sa
			1	2	3	4
5	6	7	8	9	10	11
12	13	14	15	16	17	18
19	20	21	22	23	24	25
26	27	28	29	30	31	

November

Su	Mo	Tu	We	Th	Fr	Sa
						1
2	3	4	5	6	7	8
9	10	11	12	13	14	15
16	17	18	19	20	21	22
23	24	25	26	27	28	29
30						

December

Su	Mo	Tu	We	Th	Fr	Sa
	1	2	3	4	5	6
7	8	9	10	11	12	13
14	15	16	17	18	19	20
21	22	23	24	25	26	27
28	29	30	31			

January

February

March

April

May

June

July

August

September

October

November

December

2015

January

Su	Mo	Tu	We	Th	Fr	Sa
				1	2	3
4	5	6	7	8	9	10
11	12	13	14	15	16	17
18	19	20	21	22	23	24
25	26	27	28	29	30	31

February

Su	Mo	Tu	We	Th	Fr	Sa
1	2	3	4	5	6	7
8	9	10	11	12	13	14
15	16	17	18	19	20	21
22	23	24	25	26	27	28

March

Su	Mo	Tu	We	Th	Fr	Sa
1	2	3	4	5	6	7
8	9	10	11	12	13	14
15	16	17	18	19	20	21
22	23	24	25	26	27	28
29	30	31				

April

Su	Mo	Tu	We	Th	Fr	Sa
			1	2	3	4
5	6	7	8	9	10	11
12	13	14	15	16	17	18
19	20	21	22	23	24	25
26	27	28	29	30		

May

Su	Mo	Tu	We	Th	Fr	Sa
					1	2
3	4	5	6	7	8	9
10	11	12	13	14	15	16
17	18	19	20	21	22	23
24	25	26	27	28	29	30
31						

June

Su	Mo	Tu	We	Th	Fr	Sa
	1	2	3	4	5	6
7	8	9	10	11	12	13
14	15	16	17	18	19	20
21	22	23	24	25	26	27
28	29	30				

July

Su	Mo	Tu	We	Th	Fr	Sa
			1	2	3	4
5	6	7	8	9	10	11
12	13	14	15	16	17	18
19	20	21	22	23	24	25
26	27	28	29	30	31	

August

Su	Mo	Tu	We	Th	Fr	Sa
						1
2	3	4	5	6	7	8
9	10	11	12	13	14	15
16	17	18	19	20	21	22
23	24	25	26	27	28	29
30	31					

September

Su	Mo	Tu	We	Th	Fr	Sa
		1	2	3	4	5
6	7	8	9	10	11	12
13	14	15	16	17	18	19
20	21	22	23	24	25	26
27	28	29	30			

October

Su	Mo	Tu	We	Th	Fr	Sa
				1	2	3
4	5	6	7	8	9	10
11	12	13	14	15	16	17
18	19	20	21	22	23	24
25	26	27	28	29	30	31

November

Su	Mo	Tu	We	Th	Fr	Sa
1	2	3	4	5	6	7
8	9	10	11	12	13	14
15	16	17	18	19	20	21
22	23	24	25	26	27	28
29	30					

December

Su	Mo	Tu	We	Th	Fr	Sa
		1	2	3	4	5
6	7	8	9	10	11	12
13	14	15	16	17	18	19
20	21	22	23	24	25	26
27	28	29	30	31		

January

February

March

April

May

June

July

August

September

October

November

December

1-Year Bible

Reading Schedule

1-Year Bible Reading Schedule

JANUARY

1	Genesis 1-2; Matthew 1
2	Genesis 3-5; Matthew 2
3	Genesis 6-8; Matthew 3
4	Genesis 9-11;Matthew 4
5	Genesis 12-14; Matthew 5:1-26
6	Genesis 15-17; Matthew 5:27-48
7	Genesis 18-19; Matthew 6
8	Genesis 20-22; Matthew 7
9	Genesis 23-24; Matthew 8
10	Genesis 25-26; Matthew 9:1-17
11	Genesis 27-28; Matthew 9:18-38
12	Genesis 29-30; Matthew 10: 1-23
13	Genesis 31-32; Matthew 10:24-42
14	Genesis 33-35; Matthew 11
15	Genesis 36-37; Matthew 12:1-21
16	Genesis 38-40; Matthew 12:22-50
17	Genesis 41; Matthew 13:1-32
18	Genesis 42-43; Matthew 13:33-58
19	Genesis 44-45; Matthew 14:1-21
20	Genesis 46-48; Matthew 14:22-36
21	Genesis 49-50; Matthew 15:1-20
22	Exodus 1-3; Matthew 15:21-39
23	Exodus 4-6; Matthew 16
24	Exodus 7-8; Matthew 17
25	Exodus 9-10; Matthew 18:1-20
26	Exodus 11-12; Matthew 18:21-35
27	Exodus 13-15; Matthew 19:1-15
28	Exodus 16-18; Matthew 19:16-30
29	Exodus 19-21; Matthew 20:1-16
30	Exodus 22-24; Matthew 20:17-34
31	Exodus 25-26; Matthew 21:1-22

FEBRUARY

1	Exodus 27-28; Matthew 21:23-46
2	Exodus 29-30; Matthew 22:1-22
3	Exodus 31-33; Matthew 22:23-46
4	Exodus 34-36; Matthew 23:1-22
5	Exodus 37-38; Matthew 23:23-39
6	Exodus 39-40; Matthew 24:1-22
7	Leviticus 1-3; Matthew 24:23-51
8	Leviticus 4-6; Matthew 25:1-30
9	Leviticus 7-9; Matthew 25:31-46
10	Leviticus 10-12; Matthew 26:1-19
11	Leviticus 13; Matthew 26:20-54
12	Leviticus 14; Matthew 26:55-75
13	Leviticus 15-17; Matthew 27:1-31
14	Leviticus 18-19; Matthew 27:32-66
15	Leviticus 20-21: Matthew 28
16	Leviticus 22-23; Mark 1:1-22
17	Leviticus 24-25; Mark 1:23-45
18	Leviticus 26-27; Mark 2
19	Numbers 1-2; Mark 3:1-21
20	Numbers 3-4; Mark 3:22-35
21	Numbers 5-6; Mark 4:1-20
22	Numbers 7; Mark 4:21-41
23	Numbers 8-10; Mark 5:1-20
24	Numbers 11-13; Mark 5:21-43
25	Numbers 14-15; Mark 6:1-32
26	Numbers 16-17; Mark 6:33-56
27	Numbers 18-20; Mark 7:1-13
28	Numbers 21-22; Mark 7:14-37

MARCH

1 Numbers 23-27; Mark 8:1-38
2 Numbers 28-29; Mark 9:1-29
3 Numbers 30-31; Mark 9:30-50
4 Numbers 32-33; Mark 10:1-31
5 Numbers 34-36; Mark 10:32-52
6 Deuteronomy 1-2; Mark 11:1-19
7 Deuteronomy 3-4; Mark 11:20-33
8 Deuteronomy 5-7; Mark 12:1-27
9 Deuteronomy 8-10; Mark 12:28-44
10 Deuteronomy 11-13; Mark 13:1-13
11 Deuteronomy 14-16; Mark 13:14-37
12 Deuteronomy 17-19; Mark 14:1-25
13 Deuteronomy 20-22; Mark 14:26-50
14 Deuteronomy 23-25; Mark 14:51-72
15 Deuteronomy 26-27; Mark 15:1-26
16 Deuteronomy 28; Mark 15:27-47
17 Deuteronomy 29-30; Mark 16
18 Deuteronomy 31-32; Luke 1:1-23
19 Deuteronomy 33-34; Luke 1:24-56
20 Joshua 1-3; Luke 1:57-80
21 Joshua 4-6; Luke 2:1-24
22 Joshua 7-8; Luke 2:25-52
23 Joshua 9-10; Luke 3
24 Joshua 11-13; Luke 4:1-32
25 Joshua 14-15; Luke 4:33-44
26 Joshua 16-18; Luke 5:1-16
27 Joshua 19-20; Luke 5:17-39
28 Joshua 21-22; Luke 6:1-26
29 Joshua 23-24; Luke 6:27-49
30 Judges 1-2; Luke 7:1-30
31 Judges 3-5; Luke 7:31-50

APRIL

1 Judges 6-7; Luke 8:1-21
2 Judges 8-9; Luke 8:22-56
3 Judges 10-11; Luke 9:1-36
4 Judges 12-14; Luke 9:37-62
5 Judges 15-17; Luke 10:1-24
6 Judges 18-19; Luke 10:25-42
7 Judges 20-21; Luke 11:1-28
8 Ruth: Luke 11:29-54
9 1 Samuel 1-3; Luke 12:1-34
10 1 Samuel 4-6; Luke 12:35-59
11 1 Samuel 7-9; Luke 13:1-21
12 1 Samuel 10-12; Luke 13:22-35
13 1 Samuel 13-14; Luke 14:1-24
14 1 Samuel 15-16; Luke 14:25-35
15 1 Samuel 17-18; Luke 15:1-10
16 1 Samuel 19-21; Luke 15:11-32
17 1 Samuel 22-24; Luke 16:1-18
18 1 Samuel 25-26; Luke 16:19-31
19 1 Samuel 27-29; Luke 17:1-19
20 1 Samuel 30-31; Luke 17:20-37
21 2 Samuel 1-3; Luke 18:1-17
22 2 Samuel 4-6; Luke 18:18-43
23 2 Samuel 7-9; Luke 19:1-28
24 2 Samuel 10-12; Luke 19:29-48
25 2 Samuel 13-14; Luke 20:1-26
26 2 Samuel 15-16; Luke 20:27-47
27 2 Samuel 17-18; Luke 21:1-19
28 2 Samuel 19-20; Luke 21:20-38
29 2 Samuel 21-22; Luke 22:1-30
30 2 Samuel 23-24; Luke 22:31-53

MAY

1	1 Kings 1-2; Luke 22:54-71
2	1 Kings 3-5; Luke 23:1-26
3	1 Kings 6-7; Luke 23:27-38
4	1 Kings 8-9; Luke 23:39-56
5	1 Kings 10-11; Luke 24:1-35
6	1 Kings 12-13; Luke 24:36-53
7	1 Kings 14-15; John 1:1-28
8	1 Kings 16-18; John 1:29-51
9	1 Kings 19-20; John 2
10	1 Kings 21-22; John 3:1-21
11	2 Kings 1-3; John 3:22-36
12	2 Kings 4-5; John 4:1-30
13	2 Kings 6-8; John 4:31-54
14	2 Kings 9-11; John 5:1-24
15	2 Kings 12-14; John 5:25-47
16	2 Kings 15-17; John 6:1-21
17	2 Kings 18-19; John 6:22-44
18	2 Kings 20-22; John 6:45-71
19	2 Kings 23-25; John 7:1-31
20	1 Chronicles 1-2; John 7:32-53
21	1 Chronicles 3-5; John 8:1-20
22	1 Chronicles 6-7; John 8:21-36
23	1 Chronicles 8-10; John 8:37-59
24	1 Chronicles 11-13; John 9:1-23
25	1 Chronicles 14-16; John 9:24-41
26	1 Chronicles 17-19; John 10:1-21
27	1 Chronicles 20-22; John 10:22-42
28	1 Chronicles 23-25; John 11:1-17
29	1 Chronicles 26-27; John 11:18-46
30	1 Chronicles 28-29; John 11:47-57
31	2 Chronicles 1-3; John 12:1-19

JUNE

1	2 Chronicles 4-6; John 12:20-50
2	2 Chronicles 7-9; John 13:1-17
3	2 Chronicles 10-12; John 13:18-38
4	2 Chronicles 13-16; John 14
5	2 Chronicles 17-19; John 15
6	2 Chronicles 20-22; John 16:1-15
7	2 Chronicles 23-26; John 16:16-23
8	2 Chronicles 27-28; John 17
9	2 Chronicles 29-31; John 18:1-23
10	2 Chronicles 32-33; John 18:24-40
11	2 Chronicles 34-36; John 19:1-22
12	Ezra 1-2; John 19:23-42
13	Ezra 3-5; John 20
14	Ezra 6-8; John 21
15	Ezra 9-10; Acts 1
16	Nehemiah 1-3; Acts 2:1-13
17	Nehemiah 4-6; Acts 2:14-47
18	Nehemiah 7-8; Acts 3
19	Nehemiah 9-11; Acts 4:1-22
20	Nehemiah 12-13; Acts 4:23-37
21	Esther 1-3; Acts 5:1-16
22	Esther 4-6; Acts 5:17-42
23	Esther 7-10; Acts 6
24	Job 1-3; Acts 7:1-19
25	Job 4-6; Acts 7:20-43
26	Job 7-9; Acts 7:44-60
27	Job 10-12; Acts 8:1-25
28	Job 13-15; Acts 8:26-40
29	Job 16-18; Acts 9:1-22
30	Job 19-20; Acts 9:23-43

JULY

1	Job 21-22; Acts 10:1-23
2	Job 23-25; Acts 10:24-48
3	Job 26-28; Acts 11
4	Job 29-30; Acts 12
5	Job 31-32; Acts 13:1-23
6	Job 33-34; Acts 13:24-52
7	Job 35-37; Acts 14
8	Job 38-39; Acts 15:1-21
9	Job 40-42; Acts 15:22-41
10	Psalms 1-3; Acts 16:1-15
11	Psalms 4-6; Acts 16:16-40
12	Psalms 7-9; Acts 17:1-15
13	Psalms 10-12; Acts 17:16-34
14	Psalms 13-16; Acts 18
15	Psalms 17-18; Acts 19:1-20
16	Psalms 19-21; Acts 19:21-41
17	Psalms 22-24; Acts 20:1-16
18	Psalms 25-27; Acts 20:17-38
19	Psalms 28-30; Acts 21:1-14
20	Psalms 31-33; Acts 21:15-40
21	Psalms 34-35; Acts 22
22	Psalms 36-37; Acts 23:1-11
23	Psalms 38-40; Acts 23:12-35
24	Psalms 41-43; Acts 24
25	Psalms 44-46; Acts 25
26	Psalms 47-49; Acts 26
27	Psalms 50-52; Acts 27:1-25
28	Psalms 53-55; Acts 27:26-44
29	Psalms 56-58; Acts 28:1-15
30	Psalms 59-61; Acts 28:16-31
31	Psalms 62-64; Romans 1

AUGUST

1	Psalms 65-67; Romans 2
2	Psalms 68-69; Romans 3
3	Psalms 70-72; Romans 4
4	Psalms 73-74; Romans 5
5	Psalms 75-77; Romans 6
6	Psalms 78; Romans 7
7	Psalms 79-81; Romans 8:1-18
8	Psalms 82-84; Romans 8:19-39
9	Psalms 85-87; Romans 9
10	Psalms 88-89; Romans 10
11	Psalms 90-92; Romans 11:1-21
12	Psalms 93-95; Romans 11:22-36
13	Psalms 96-98; Romans 12
14	Psalms 99-102; Romans 13
15	Psalms 103-104; Romans 14
16	Psalms 105-106; Romans 15:1-20
17	Psalms 107-108; Romans 15:21-33
18	Psalms 109-111; Romans 16
19	Psalms 112-115; 1 Corinthians 1
20	Psalms 116-118; 1 Corinthians 2
21	Psalms 119:1-48; 1 Corinthians 3
22	Psalms 119:49-104; 1 Corinthians 4
23	Psalms 119:105-176; 1 Corinthians 5
24	Psalms 120-123; 1 Corinthians 6
25	Psalms 124-127; 1 Corinthians 7:1-24
26	Psalms 128-131; 1 Corinthians 7:25-40
27	Psalms 132-135; 1 Corinthians 8
28	Psalms 136-138; 1 Corinthians 9
29	Psalms 139-141; 1 Corinthians 10:1-13
30	Psalms 142-144; 1 Corinthians 10:14-33
31	Psalms 145-147; 1 Corinthians 11:1-15

SEPTEMBER

1 Psalms 148-150; 1 Corinthians 11:16-34
2 Proverbs 1-2; 1 Corinthians 12
3 Proverbs 3-4; 1 Corinthians 13
4 Proverbs 5-6; 1 Corinthians 14:1-20
5 Proverbs 7-8; 1 Corinthians 14:21-40
6 Proverbs 9-10; 1 Corinthians 15;1-32
7 Proverbs 11-12; 1 Corinthians 15:33-58
8 Proverbs 13-14; 1 Corinthians 16
9 Proverbs 15-16; 2 Corinthians 1
10 Proverbs 17-18; 2 Corinthians 2
11 Proverbs 19-20; 2 Corinthians 3
12 Proverbs 21-22; 2 Corinthians 4
13 Proverbs 23-24; 2 Corinthians 5
14 Proverbs 25-27; 2 Corinthians 6
15 Proverbs 28-29; 2 Corinthians 7
16 Proverbs 30-31; 2 Corinthians 8
17 Ecclesiastes 1-3; 2 Corinthians 9
18 Ecclesiastes 4-6; 2 Corinthians 10
19 Ecclesiastes 7-9; 2 Corinthians 11:1-15
20 Ecclesiastes 10-12; 2 Corinthians 11:16-33
21 Song of Solomon 1-3; 2 Corinthians 12
22 Song of Solomon 4-5; 2 Corinthians 13
23 Song of Solomon 6-8; Galatians 1
24 Isaiah 1-3; Galatians 2
25 Isaiah 4-6; Galatians 3
26 Isaiah 7-9; Galatians 4
27 Isaiah 10-12; Galatians 5
28 Isaiah 13-15; Galatians 6
29 Isaiah 16-18; Ephesians 1
30 Isaiah 19-21; Ephesians 2

OCTOBER

1 Isaiah 22-23; Ephesians 3
2 Isaiah 24-26; Ephesians 4
3 Isaiah 27-28; Ephesians 5
4 Isaiah 29-30; Ephesians 6
5 Isaiah 31-33; Philippians 1
6 Isaiah 34-36; Philippians 2
7 Isaiah 37-38; Philippians 3
8 Isaiah 39-40; Philippians 4
9 Isaiah 41-42; Colossians 1
10 Isaiah 43-44; Colossians 2
11 Isaiah 45-47; Colossians 3
12 Isaiah 48-49; Colossians 4
13 Isaiah 50-52; 1 Thessalonians 1
14 Isaiah 53-55; 1 Thessalonians 2
15 Isaiah 56-58; 1 Thessalonians 3
16 Isaiah 59-61; 1 Thessalonians 4
17 Isaiah 62-64; 1 Thessalonians 5
18 Isaiah 65-66; 2 Thessalonians 1
19 Jeremiah 1-2; 2 Thessalonians 2
20 Jeremiah 3-4; 2 Thessalonians 3
21 Jeremiah 5-6; 1 Timothy 1
22 Jeremiah 7-8; 1 Timothy 2
23 Jeremiah 9-10; 1 Timothy 3
24 Jeremiah 11-13; 1 Timothy 4
25 Jeremiah 14-16; 1 Timothy 5
26 Jeremiah 17-19; 1 Timothy 6
27 Jeremiah 20-22; 2 Timothy 1
28 Jeremiah 23-24; 2 Timothy 2
29 Jeremiah 25-26; 2 Timothy 3
30 Jeremiah 27-28; 2 Timothy 4
31 Jeremiah 29-30; Titus 1

NOVEMBER

1 Jeremiah 31-32; Titus 2
2 Jeremiah 33-35; Titus 3
3 Jeremiah 36-37; Philemon
4 Jeremiah 38-39; Hebrews 1
5 Jeremiah 40-42; Hebrews 2
6 Jeremiah 43-45; Hebrews 3
7 Jeremiah 46-48; Hebrews 4
8 Jeremiah 49-50; Hebrews 5
9 Jeremiah 51-52; Hebrews 6
10 Lamentations 1-2; Hebrews 7
11 Lamentations 3-5; Hebrews 8
12 Ezekiel 1-3; Hebrews 9
13 Ezekiel 4-6; Hebrews 10:1-23
14 Ezekiel 7-9; Hebrews 10:24-39
15 Ezekiel 10-12; Hebrews 11:1-19
16 Ezekiel 13-15; Hebrews 11:20-40
17 Ezekiel 16; Hebrews 12
18 Ezekiel 17-19; Hebrews 13
19 Ezekiel 20-21; James 1
20 Ezekiel 22-23; James 2
21 Ezekiel 24-26; James 3
22 Ezekiel 27-28; James 4
23 Ezekiel 29-31; James 5
24 Ezekiel 32-33; 1 Peter 1
25 Ezekiel 34-35; 1 Peter 2
26 Ezekiel 36-37; 1 Peter 3
27 Ezekiel 38-39; 1 Peter 4
28 Ezekiel 40; 1 Peter 5
29 Ezekiel 41-42; 2 Peter 1
30 Ezekiel 43-44; 2 Peter 2

DECEMBER

1 Ezekiel 45-46; 2 Peter 3
2 Ezekiel 47-48; 1 John 1
3 Daniel 1-2; 1 John 2
4 Daniel 3-4; 1 John 3
5 Daniel 5-6; 1 John 4
6 Daniel 7-8; 1 John 5
7 Daniel 9-10; 2 John
8 Daniel 11-12; 3 John
9 Hosea 1-4; Jude
10 Hosea 5-8; Revelation 1
11 Hosea 9-11; Revelation 2
12 Hosea 12-14; Revelation 3
13 Joel; Revelation 4
14 Amos 1-3; Revelation 5
15 Amos 4-6; Revelation 6
16 Amos 7-9; Revelation 7
17 Obadiah; Revelation 8
18 Jonah; Revelation 9
19 Micah 1-3; Revelation 10
20 Micah 4-5; Revelation 11
21 Micah 6-7; Revelation 12
22 Nahum; Revelation 13
23 Habakkuk; Revelation 14
24 Zephaniah; Revelation 15
25 Haggai; Revelation 16
26 Zechariah 1-3; Revelation 17
27 Zechariah 4-6; Revelation 18
28 Zechariah 7-9; Revelation 19
29 Zechariah 10-12; Revelation 20
30 Zechariah 13-14; Revelation 21
31 Malachi; Revelation 22

Contact Information

If you would like to correspond with Dr. Landry, book speaking engagements or attend a *Caregivers Speak* meeting, please write us at:

glandrybook@gmail.com

To order additional copies of this book visit:

www.caregiversspeaks.org

Made in United States
Cleveland, OH
04 November 2026

47647255R00147